AQUAEROBICS, SR.®
Easy Pool Exercises for Seniors

by Dorothy V. Kelly

TOP OF THE MOUNTAIN PUBLISHING
Largo, Florida 34643-5117 U.S.A.

TOP OF THE MOUNTAIN PUBLISHING
11701 South Belcher Road, Suite #123
Largo, Florida 34643-5117 U.S.A. SAN 287-590X
FAX (813) 536-3681 PHONE (813) 530-0110

Copyright 1993 by Dorothy V. Kelly

Library of Congress Cataloging in Publication Data
Kelly, Dorothy V.,
Aquaerobics, Sr. : easy pool exercises for seniors / by Dorothy V. Kelly.
p.cm.
ISBN 1-56087-039-7 : $12.95
1. Aquatic exercises. 2. Exercise for the aged. I. Title.
GV838.53.E94K45 1993 613.7'16–dc20   93-17459 CIP

Cover Design and Illustrations by Stan Morrison

Manufactured in the United States of America

TABLE OF CONTENTS

To Whom It May Concern:

Three years ago I suffered a stroke, partially losing the use of my left arm and leg. Each morning, for the next two winters, I joined a group who exercised in the pool and found it to be very helpful in my recovery.

This group was organized by Dorothy Kelly, who did an excellent job keeping us all interested!

Sincerely,
Harry "Buddy" Sweet
Pointe West Park, Largo, Florida

FOREWORD

Author Dorothy Kelly's timing is perfect! *Aquaerobics, Sr.®: Easy Pool Exercises for Seniors* is exactly what the public, and especially senior citizens, need to become aware of and practice. *Aquaerobics, Sr.®* is in the forefront of the latest trend—SAFE exercising.

This is a book that can definitely DE-CREASE my chiropractic practice. Why would I write a foreword for it? Well, it's too good to hide. Exercises and techniques in *Aquaerobics, Sr.®* have been especially designed to help individuals, especially seniors, who want a no-nonsense, physical cardiovascular work-out without the high potential for injury. These exercises can be performed by people with arthritis, as a physical therapy method, or to assist in flexibility. Here is an easy-to-follow program for individuals trying to shed extra weight. It also can be a stress reliever and to strengthen back muscles.

All too often, my patients come in with torn ligaments, aching muscles and broken bones sustained from exercise and/or sports-related injuries that could have been avoided had they chosen activities more suited to their body, health and age. Many of my patients are seniors who complain about their efforts of trying to maintain a physically fit body, but who find aerobic activity (such as running, jogging, walking and actual aerobic classes) too strenuous and painful.

If you're thinking to yourself, "I'm past the age where exercise will do any good," or "Any type of exercise is painful," or "It's no fun to exercise," then *Aquaerobics, Sr.®* is definitely the book for you! Staying fit and healthy is every bit as necessary when we mature as when we are younger. My patients often think that being seniors means giving up on body maintenance. Why? They claim a lack of mobility, endurance, ability and motivation.

They claim exercising isn't FUN and EASY with maturity.

Well, I let these patients in on the latest secret...Ms. Kelly has proven exercising is not only a fitness "thing," it is also a focal point for soothing the mind and socializing. As we age, we must keep our bodies fit, maintain good health and stay youthful in our mind and our physique. Everything we put into our minds and bodies in the form of thoughts, food and drink, will surely reflect itself in our overall health and fitness. Pool exercising is a way to maintain strength, muscle tone, and endurance. It's a great way to relieve mental stress. This book also has over 60 positive statements to help develop and maintain a positive outlook, motivate you and soothe your mind!

With *Aquaerobics, Sr.*®, you will be able to exercise in a group environment to techniques which have been proven safe and effective. It's usually difficult to begin, but Ms. Kelly's pool exercises allows you to invite your friends to join in on spending some "fun time," in the pool you've not used since the kids have left home. It's an easy way for building and maintaining a good physique! For the over-40 crowd, hard bodies are out; good, healthful bodies are in.

This book also comes complete with easy-to-follow text, graphics and my fitness explanations as to which areas of your body the various movements will benefit. *Aquaerobics, Sr.*® may decrease my business, but it will surely increase your health and fitness. After all, isn't that what happy and complete living is all about? Have fun...be safe...and wear some sun screen to protect your youthful glow!

Dr. Robert Malone,
D.C., D.A.C.T.S., D.C.C.T.

Dr. Robert Malone has over 26-years of clinical experience in chiropractic medicine. He is a 1967 graduate of The Palmer College of Chiropractic, with post-graduate study in Orthopedics and Disability Evaluation. He is a certified lecturer at the Life College, Post-Graduate Studies on Thermography. Dr. Malone is also on the teaching staffs of A.C.T.S. (American Chiropractic Thermographic Society) and I.C.A. College of Thermography.

He is active in several clinical chiropractic organizations, including: I.C.A.; the Florida Chiropractic Society; A.C.T.S. (American Chiropractic Thermographic Society); and I.A.C.T. (International Asociation of Chiropractic Thermology). He is currently practicing chiropractic medicine in Largo, Florida, and holds active licenses in both Florida and Mississippi.

Along with his professional career, Dr. Malone believes in a well-rounded lifestyle of healthy eating, exercising and mental fitness. He lives in Clearwater, Florida with his wife, Wanda, and their three children.

INTRODUCTION

Water exercises are the easiest and most effective exercises for stiff and aching muscles, as you have the buoyancy of the water to help you. This book contains exercises for every part of your body: head, neck, shoulders, arms, hands, fingers, bust, stomach, hips, thighs, legs, knees, ankles and even your toes. Some are for balance, twisting, bending and stretching. Try to do some every day, or at least three times a week, and remember to inhale and exhale *deeply* while performing these exercises. You do not have to be a swimmer, as most of these exercises can be done in shallow water. (You must for safety reasons, however, be able to swim to do the deep water exercises.) Try to get the men into the water — the exercises are just as good for them, too!

Aerobic exercise is too strenuous and fast for us seniors to do. We can, however, keep up by doing the exercises written in this up-to-date book. You should not rush through the activities; doing them too fast will not help. These exercises are a must for arthritic patients and for those with broken bones (upon your doctor's approval). You are advised not to perform these exercises individually — it's always more motivating, safer (and seemingly easier!) as a group effort. There are many exercises to choose from. If you have a leader, he or she can coordinate which exercises to practice. It is better to start with a few exercises and increase the number as you feel everyone is able to do more. Enjoy this fun, safe and easy-to-move method of exercise!

Some Things to Remember

A. Never roll your shoulders forward when you do the shoulder exercises, roll your shoulders backward only (as seniors are inclined to be round-shouldered). This will help in your keeping correct and healthy posture.

B. Keep your fingers open when doing arm or hand exercises, so the water will flow through your fingers. This position will ease any pain in your fingers.

C. Do your head exercises slowly, so you won't get dizzy.

D. Never roll your head around in a circle, as you have many little bones in the back of your neck which you may injure their alignment.

E. Do not force yourself to do any exercise which causes pain or discomfort. Let it go, and try it again the next day, until you can do it without it hurting. Be sure to consult a physician if you experience unbearable pain. Remember, it is better to play it safe, rather than over-exert yourself!

F. Do not exercise in the pool alone, have a friend over to exercise with you or someone by the pool while you exercise.

The entire exercise program will take about *seventy minutes* to do. There are forty-three exercises which can be done in shallow water. Taller people should go out deeper and save the shallow places for the shorter individuals. There are nineteen exercises to do in deep water, which are intended to tighten leg and stomach muscles, and help in flexibility. You can do them in as deep of water as you can stand and still maintain your head above the water.

GROUP CLASSES

TO BEGIN: A good way to start the class is to form a circle. The person to the right of the leader will say, "Good Morning, I'm Cora-1." Then, "I'm Dot-2." Next, "I'm Kay-3." This activity will allow you to learn all the names and the numbers in the group.

DURING CLASS: Do not allow talking during the exercises. Take a rest about halfway through, then get back to serious business.

TO END: End the class with the "Hokey Pokey," so all members will be exercising their shoulders, arms, feet and hips, and will have fun singing the song as they do it. Here is another song you might try at closing, sung to the tune of "Ach Der Lieber Augustin." Have your class members form a circle with their arms around the backs of their neighbors. Then move around to the left, while singing the first verse, and to the right as all sing the second verse.

SING ALONG

The   more   we   get   together,
together, together,
The   more   we   get   together,
the happier we'll be.
For your friends are my friends, and
my friends are your friends.
The   more   we   get   together
the happier we'll be.

The   more   we   get   together,
together, together,
The   more   we   get   together
the healthier we'll be.

For your friends are my friends, and
my friends are your friends.
The   more   we   get   together
the healthier we'll be.

You may have your own ideas for a closing song, and the others may suggest something which will be fun. Build a lively, entertaining atmosphere, and the group will want to come back!

A Poem For Dottie

Whether exercise or aquacise
or dancing in a line,
The hours you devote daily,
add up to a lot of time.

We stretch, and roll,
and grunt and gasp,
Eat all the more,
and forget to fast.

But we're having fun,
and all feel fit,
And do appreciate
your special part in it.

So please accept this little gift,
We hope it will your spirits lift,
We love you and appreciate
your faithfulness which is so great.

Peg

HEALTH DISCLAIMER

The swimming exercises discussed in this book are intended as part of an overall exercise program. They can be performed in place of aerobic activity, especially for seniors who find aerobics too strenuous.

It is important to remember any change in physical activity or any exericse program should be taken under the direction of your doctor. All forms of physical exercise should be practiced under safe and regulated conditions. At no time should these pool exercises be performed under physical distress or pain. Supervision is recommended at all times — whether it is with a group or as an individual. If pain or discomfort results from exercising, immediately cease activity and consult a physician. Notify your doctor *before you begin* your exercise program. If your doctor has any questions, have your doctor call us at 813 530-0110 for a complementery professional copy of this book.

> ## PLEASE NOTE:
>
> When exercises are performed out-of-doors,
> sunscreen is recommended.
> Exercise in the cooler morning hours or late in the afternoon.
> Avoid exercising in the direct sun between 11 A.M.
> and 2 P.M.

Warm up with...

SHALLOW WATER EXERCISES

"Friendship is one mind in two bodies."

Mencius

HEALTH & FITNESS NOTES

1. BALLET WARM UP:

This exercise loosens and warms up the shoulders, elbows, upper and lower back. It also gets the circulation flowing!

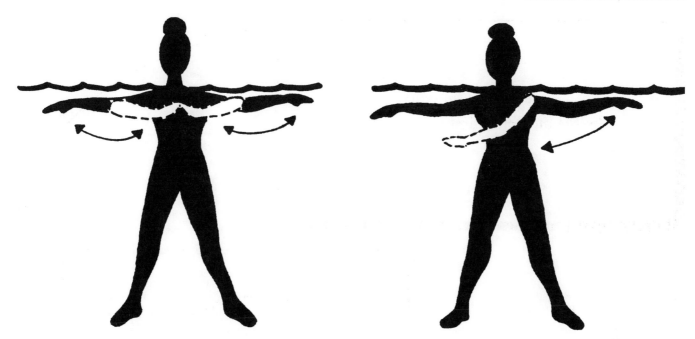

1. BALLET WARM UP:

With arms slightly under water, swing both arms to your chest. Swing both arms outward to the sides, swing Right arm across to the Left around your Left knee.

Swing Right arm back, around Right knee. Swing Left arm down around Right knee, swing Left arm over around Left knee. Repeat 5 times.

"...the one who wins,
is the one who thinks they can."

O.P. Ghai

HEALTH & FITNESS NOTES

2. ROLLY POLLY:
Loosens and adds flexibility to the wrists.

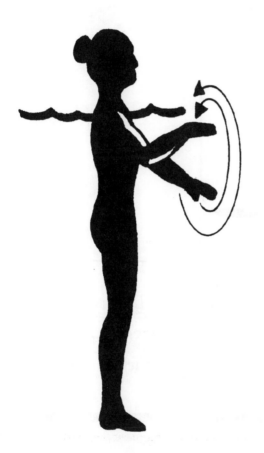

2. ROLLY POLLY:

With arms under water a little lower than your chest, roll hands over each other with your fingers open. Roll 20 times, reverse and roll 20 more.

"Friends, though absent, are still present."

Marcus Cicero

HEALTH & FITNESS NOTES

3. ARM SCISSORS:
This exercise flexes the shoulders.

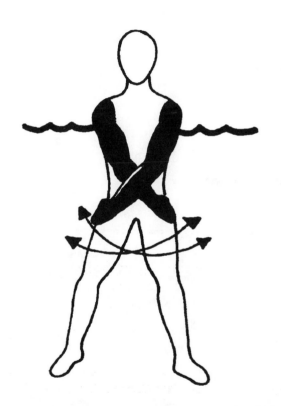

3. ARM SCISSORS:

With both arms hanging at your sides, criss-cross your arms across your chest as you bring them to the top of the water. Criss-cross them as you swing them back down and up to the top of the water. Repeat 10 times. Do the same placing your arms in back of you.

"*The further I advance in life, the more convinced I am of the necessity of that principle of wisdom which befits our nature: enjoy what lies in your own hands.*"

Eugene Delacroix

HEALTH & FITNESS NOTES

4. HANDS OVER:

4A loosens and exercises the wrists and upper forearms.
4B mobilizes the shoulder joints.

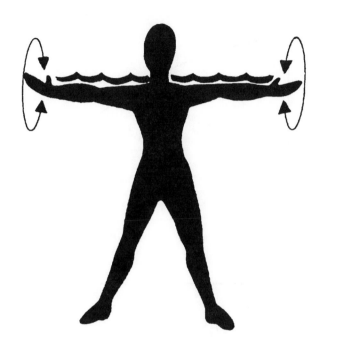 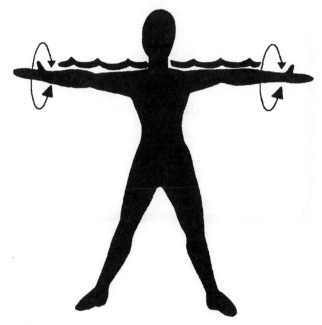

4. HANDS OVER:

A. Stretch arms out to the sides just a little under water with palms facing upward. Turn the palms of your hands over, and back. Repeat 20 times.

B. While arms are stretched out at your sides a little under water, make little circles with both hands 20 times (using wrist action). Reverse motion and do 20 more.

"*Success cannot be copied—cannot be successfully imitated. It is an orginial force—an individual creation.*"

Aldous Huxley

HEALTH & FITNESS NOTES

4C flexes the fingers. Especially good for arthritic fingers and hands. 4D loosens and exercises the wrists.

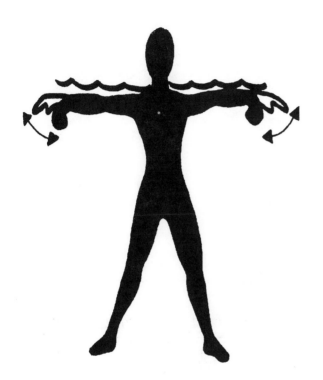

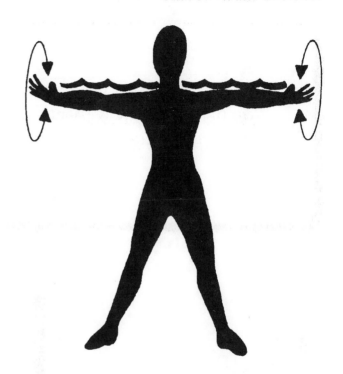

C. With your arms stretched out to the side a little under water, make a fist, stretch your fingers out as you open your hands. Repeat 20 times.

D. With your arms stretched out to the side under water, twist your wrists over and back. Twist 20 times with your fingers open.

"Practice "maketh one perfect"; and continued practice is essential to keep up that perfection."

Walter Malone

HEALTH & FITNESS NOTES

5. PUSH UPS:
Mobilizes the shoulder joints and exercises upper back muscles. This exercise should be done gently and never forced.

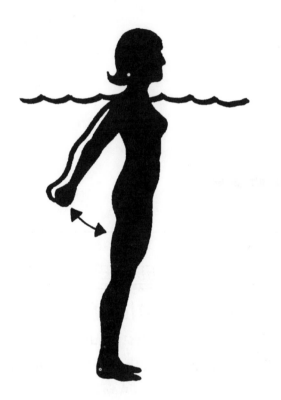

5. PUSH UPS:

Clasp your hands together in back at your buttocks, push both arms away and upward as far as you can. Go back down to the your tush. Repeat 10 times.

"That which is striking and beautiful is not always good, but that which is good is always beautiful."

Ninon de Lenclos

HEALTH & FITNESS NOTES

6. UP TO SHOULDERS:

Mobilizes the shoulder joints and exercises upper back muscles. Includes some upper arm muscle activity. Again, this exercise should be done gently and never forced.

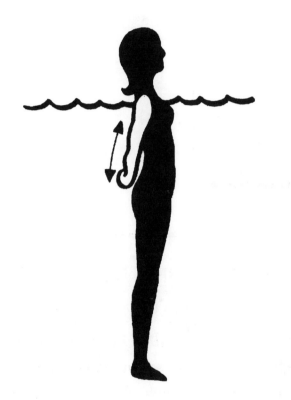

6. UP TO SHOULDERS:

Clasp your hands at the base of your spine, push both arms up to your shoulder blades (keep standing tall). Then push them down to the base of your spine. Repeat 10 times.

"The beautiful attracts the beautiful."

Leigh Hunt

HEALTH & FITNESS NOTES

7. ARMS OVER:
A good, general warm up and flexibility exercise for shoulders and lower back.

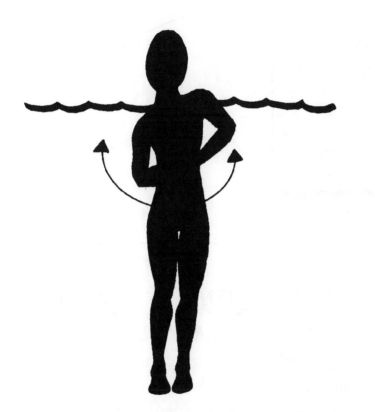

7. ARMS OVER:

Clasp your arms together at the arch in your back, swing both arms to the Right and to the Left. Repeat 20 times.

"*Happiness is a state-of-mind wherein you have found peace and fulfillment.*"

Robert Louis Stevenson

HEALTH & FITNESS NOTES

8. SHOULDER ROLL:
Very good for mobilizing shoulder joints and upper back. This exercise also works some neck muscles.

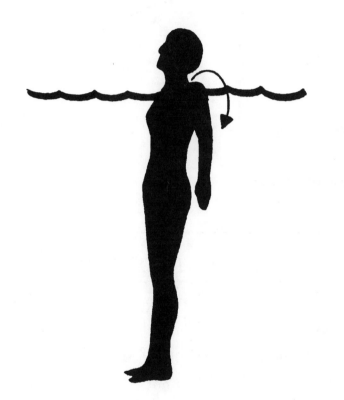

8. SHOULDER ROLL:

Roll your Right shoulder backward in a circle keeping your shoulder under water, roll 15 times. Roll your Left shoulder backward 15 times. Roll both shoulders backward together 15 times.

"To have joy one must share it —
Happiness was born a twin."

Lord Byron

HEALTH & FITNESS NOTES

9. SWING OVER HEAD:
Stretches shoulder and side muscles. It
exercises shoulder joints and elbows.
Arthritic shoulders may not like this exercise.
Do it gently and do not strain.

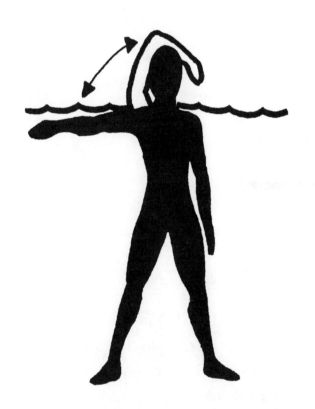

9. SWING OVER HEAD:

Touch your Right shoulder with your fingers on your Right hand, swing your Right arm over your head, touch your Left shoulder. Swing your arm back, touch your Right shoulder with your Right hand, stretch your Right arm out and touch the water with the fingers on your Right hand. Repeat 15 times. Reverse and do 15 times with your Left arm.

*"Happiness must be sipped,
not drained from life in great gulps."*

Aldous Huxley

HEALTH & FITNESS NOTES

10. SWIM BREASTSTROKE:
*Tones upper chest muscles, stretches
and exercises the shoulders.
A good loosening up exercise.*

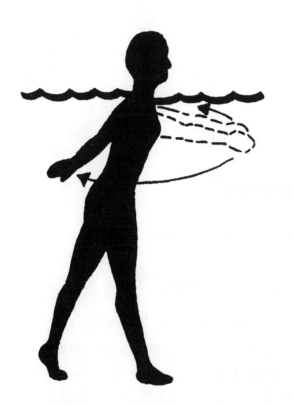

10. SWIM BREASTSTROKE:

Stretch both arms out in front a little under water. At the same time, swing Right arm to the Right side, swing Left arm to the Left side. Swing both arms back to the front, close your fists and pull your arms to your hips. Repeat 10 times.

"The deed is everything, the glory naught."

Goethe

HEALTH & FITNESS NOTES

11. STRETCH ARMS:

This is a nice little exercise that almost anyone can do for upper body and wrist workout. It also mobilizes the shoulders.

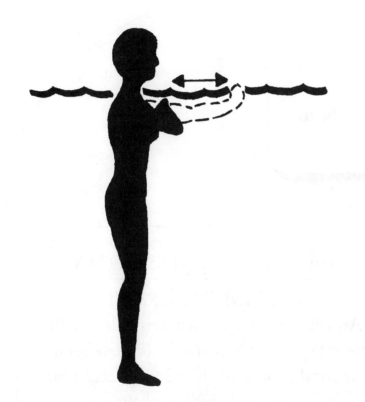

11. STRETCH ARMS:

Stretch both arms forward keeping your fingers locked loosely. Pull your arms back to your chest. Push your arms forward, then pull them back to your chest. Repeat 10 times. (Inhale as you pull your arms inward and exhale as you push your arms outward.)

"*Happiness lies, first of all, in health.*"

George William Curtis

HEALTH & FITNESS NOTES

12. STANDING CRAWL:

Arthritic or injured shoulders will benefit from this exercise. It should be done gently but firmly. Good for rotator cuff exercising and upper body workout.

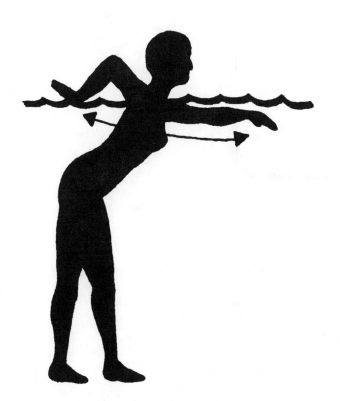

12. STANDING CRAWL:

Stand in the same place with both feet flat on the bottom of the pool. Reaching out with your Left hand, getting a "grip" on the water, pressing downward and pulling, bring your Left hand through to the thigh. Repeat, alternatively, with your Right hand. Do the Standing Crawl 30 times. (See diagram for best demonstration.)

"Life is worthwhile if you are progressing in truth and righteousness."

St. Augustine

HEALTH & FITNESS NOTES

13. SWING FISTS:
This exercise works the elbows and tones the backs of the arms.

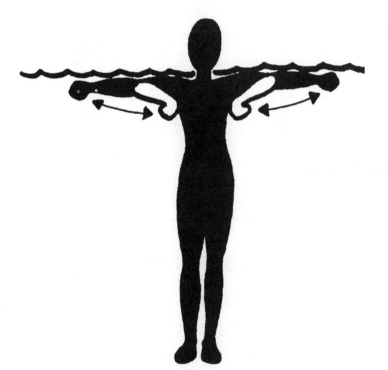

13. SWING FISTS:

Close your fists under your arm pits. Stretch your arms out to the sides, swing them back under your arm pits, swing them out to the sides, keep fists closed. Repeat 20 times.

"*A minute's success pays the failure of years.*"

Robert Browning

HEALTH & FITNESS NOTES

14. WALK:
A good workout for the ankles
and calves of the legs.

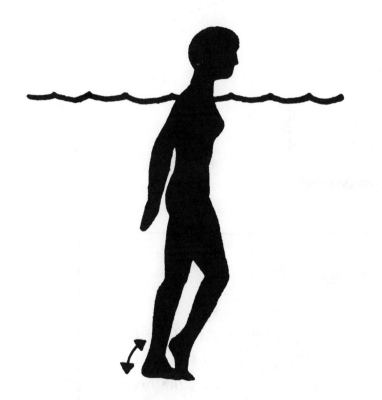

14. WALK:

Go up on the ball of your Left foot while flat on the Right foot, slightly bending the knees. Go up on the ball of your Right foot while flat on your Left foot, alternating Right and Left. Repeat 30 times.

"*Cheerfulness is a valuable success asset. It's the greatest tonic in the world for both mind and body.*"

Ralph Waldo Emerson

HEALTH & FITNESS NOTES

15. UP ON TOES:

A more strenuous workout for the ankles and calves. Do this gently and do not land hard on the heels.

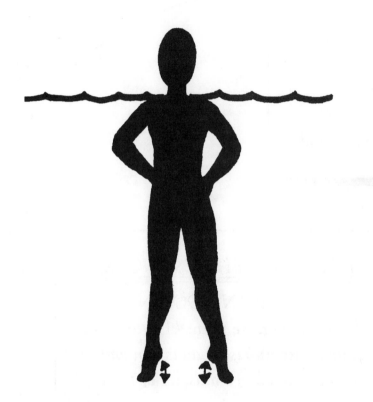

15. UP ON TOES:

Go up on the balls of both feet, stay there and balance for the count of 10. Go down flat on both feet. Repeat 5 times. Be careful, if sharp pain occurs, immediately release the tiptoes.

"*Love is not something to argue,*
reason and bargain about.
It is something to give — to feel."

Ayn Rand

HEALTH & FITNESS NOTES

16. UP AND DOWN:

Easier to balance than #15, and not
quite as strenuous. It adds workout to
the knees and large muscles of the legs.

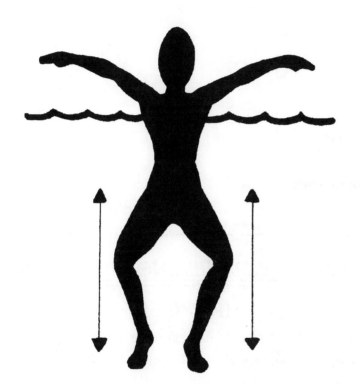

16. UP AND DOWN:

Go up on the balls of both feet, bend your knees outward as you go down in a squatting position. Go back up still on the balls of both feet, go down flat on both feet. Repeat 10 times.

"The great acts of love are done by those who habitually perform small acts of kindness."

Unknown

HEALTH & FITNESS NOTES

17. JUMP UPS:
A moderately strenuous exercise that should be done gently until it is proven that it can be done without pain. If pain develops, stop immediately.

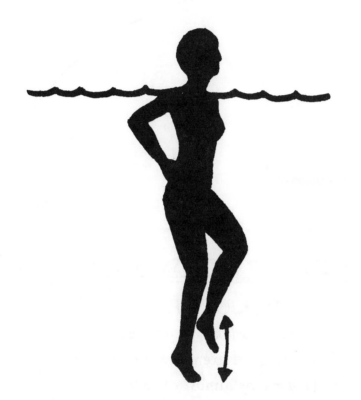

17. JUMP UPS:

Jump up on the ball of your Right foot, go down on your Right foot, push up with your Right foot and transfer onto the ball of your Left foot, go down flat on your Left foot. Push up with your Left foot then over onto the ball of your Right foot, go down flat on your Right foot. Alternate 30 times.

"It's a funny thing about life:
If you refuse to accept anything
but the best, you very often get it."

W. Somerset Maugham

HEALTH & FITNESS NOTES

18. KICK UPS:
A gentle workout for the legs.
This is a good exercise that can
be done by almost anyone.

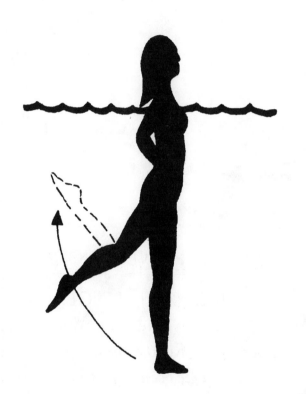

18. KICK UPS:

Kick up in back as high as you can with your Right leg. Kick up in back as high as you can with your Left leg, slightly bending your knees. Alternate and repeat 30 times.

"He most lives who thinks most,
feels the noblest, acts the best."

Bailey

HEALTH & FITNESS NOTES

19. SIDEWAYS LUNGE:

Put your hands on your hips. With legs apart, bend your Right knee down to the Right on an angle, bend your Left knee down to the Left on an angle. Repeat to the Right and to the Left 30 times.

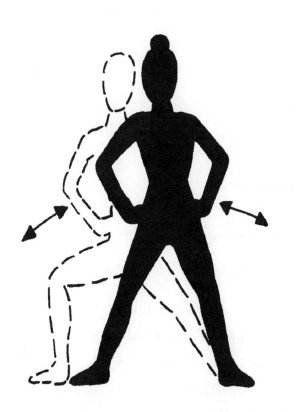

19. SIDEWAYS LUNGE:

Start with Right leg forward, bend Right knee to a 90º angle in a lunge position. Alternate with Left leg forward, and lunge to a 90º angle. Repeat and alternate 30 times.

"*Learn wisdom from the experience of others, and from their failings you will be able to correct your own faults.*"

Dandemis

HEALTH & FITNESS NOTES

20. FAST JOG:
This is one of the best cardiovascular exercises. Use common sense, as with any other exercise. If it strains you too much, don't do it.

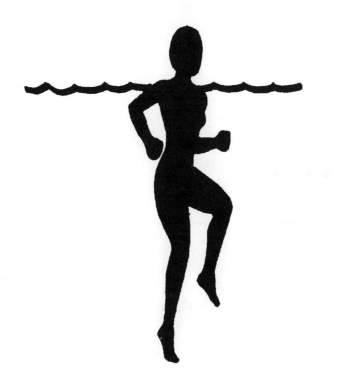

20. FAST JOG:

Run fast in place, count to 100.

"*I have only managed to live so long by carrying no hatreds.*"

Sir Winston Churchill

HEALTH & FITNESS NOTES

21. GOOSE STEP:
This exercise nicely works out the hips, upper legs and thighs.

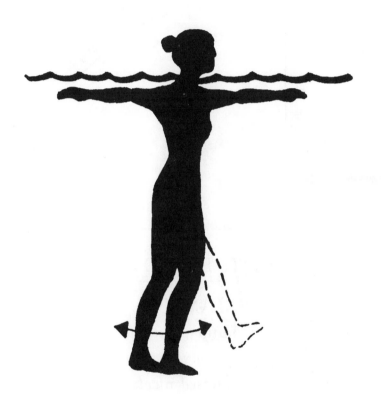

21. GOOSE STEP:

Kick your Right leg out forward and as you bring it back, kick your Left leg forward. Alternate Right and Left 30 times. (Like a German soldier march.)

Hint: You may place the palms of your hands on the lower portion of your back to ease the stress on your back while doing this exercise.

"...one should have in youth the experience
of advanced years, and in old age
the vigor of youth."

Stanislaus

HEALTH & FITNESS NOTES

22. LEG BALANCE:
This takes coordination, but once
mastered, the lower body, legs and
ankles can be exercised nicely.

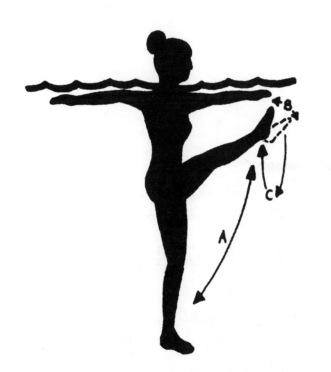

22. LEG BALANCE:

Kick your Right leg up to the top of the water or as high as you can, balance on your Left leg and count to 10. Maintain this position and flip your Right ankle up and down, 10 times. Then make a small circle with your Right foot, turning your foot to the Right 10 times. Make a circle with your Right foot turning your foot to the Left 10 times. Repeat same steps with your Left leg and foot.

"Some books are to be tasted, others to be swallowed, and some few to be chewed and digested."

Francis Bacon

HEALTH & FITNESS NOTES

23. KNEE BALANCE:
This exercise gently stretches the lower back, tones the lower abdomen and loosens the hip joints.

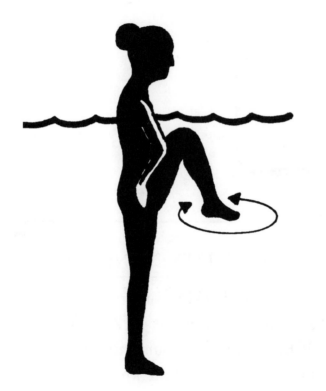

23. KNEE BALANCE:

Put your Right knee up as high as possible close to your chest, hold there and count to 10. Keep your Right knee up and make a large circle to the right with your Right calf 10 times. Then reverse the motion and make 10 more large circles. Do the same exercise with your Left calf and knee. (Similar to the "can-can" dance.)

"*Use your time wisely. Don't be a timewaster; use it for self-improvement, use it to broaden your horizons.*"

Charles Dickens

HEALTH & FITNESS NOTES

24. TUMMY IN:
Essentially the same as #12 of the DEEP WATER section, but adds isometric exercising of the upper chest.

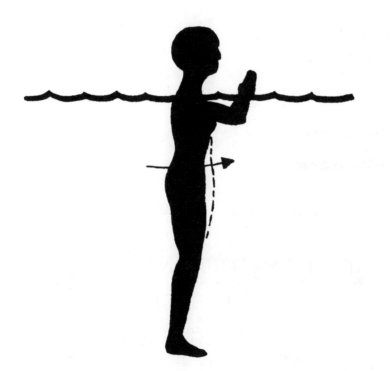

24. TUMMY IN:

Pull your stomach and derriere in tight. Press your hands together like praying, tilt your pelvis forward. Do all movements at the same time, hold in tight and count to 10. Relax, then repeat 5 times.

"*The man who lives in the present, forgetful of the past and indifferent to the future, is the man of wisdom.*"

Lord Avebury

HEALTH & FITNESS NOTES

25. CHEST BOUNCE:
Strengthens and tones the upper chest muscles.

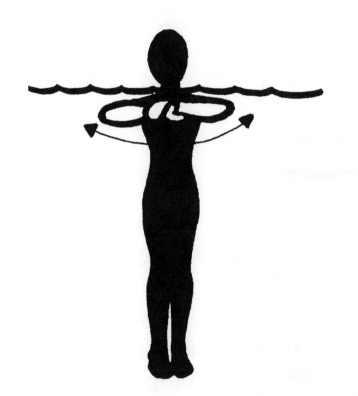

25. CHEST BOUNCE:

Cross your hands over each other, clasp your Left hand on the forearm of the Right arm, clasp your Right hand on the forearm of the Left arm. Push both hands toward your elbows at the same time. Tighten your chest/bust muscles at the same time. Repeat 20 times. (Similar to the "bust developer exercise.")

"When you look at yourself,
reflections of the ones you love
are clear for all to see."

John Anderson

HEALTH & FITNESS NOTES

26. FROGGIE:
(Same as #11 of DEEP WATER
exercises.) Primarily a leg joint exercise,
but it also tones up the lateral thighs.

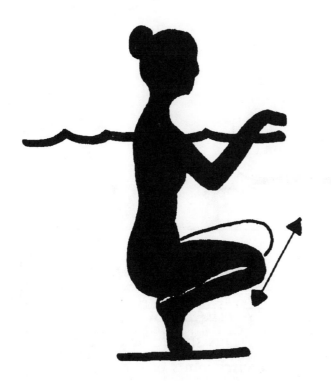

26. FROGGIE:

In a squatting position and on the balls of both feet, throw your knees outward like a frog, bring them back to the center. Touch your knees together, throw them outward again, bring them back, touch them together. Repeat 20 times.

"*Rings and jewels are not gifts,*
but apologies for gifts.
The only gift is a portion of thyself."

Emerson

HEALTH & FITNESS NOTES

27. HEAD TWIST:
27A and B. This should be done gently.
It exercises joints of the neck.

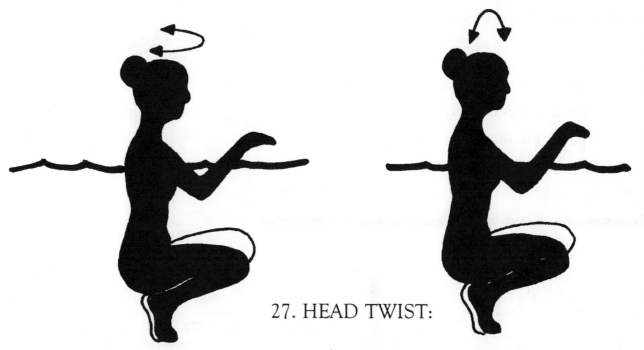

27. HEAD TWIST:

A. Squat down so only your head is out of the water, turn your head to the Right, turn your head to the Left. Repeat 20 times.

B. Bend your head to the Right, try to touch your Right shoulder with your ear. Bend your head to the Left, try to touch your Left shoulder with your ear. Repeat 20 times.

73

"*Love is of all the passions the strongest,*
for it attacks simultaneously the head,
the heart and the senses."

Voltaire

HEALTH & FITNESS NOTES

27. HEAD TWIST:
27C and D. This should be done gently.
It exercises joints of the neck.

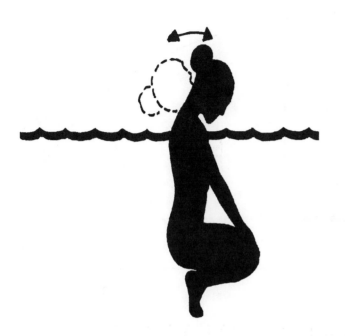

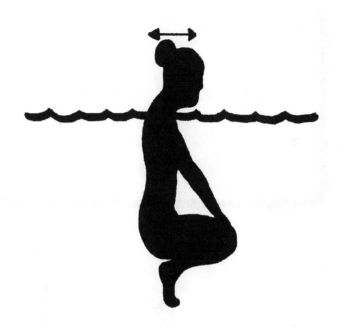

C. Bend your head straight back, touch the center of your shoulders. Bend your head forward, touch the center of your chest with your chin. Repeat 20 times.

D. Stretch your head forward with your chin skimming the water, pull your head back skimming the water. Repeat 20 times.
(Like a chicken's head movement.)

75

"*If you want to make the world a better place, take a look at yourself and make a change.*"

Michael Jackson

HEALTH & FITNESS NOTES

27. HEAD TWIST:
27E is for the "double chin."

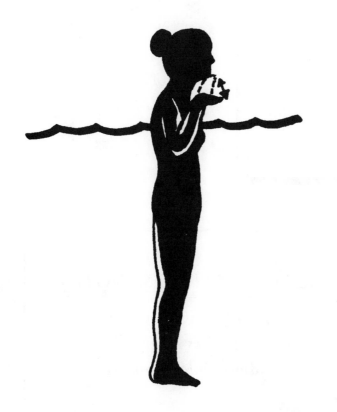

E. Slap under your chin with the back of your Right hand moving your hand from one side of the chin to the other as you gently slap.

"*Let simplicity govern your life.*"

O.P. Ghai

HEALTH & FITNESS NOTES

28. LEG SCISSORS:
This gives a gentle cardiovascular workout.

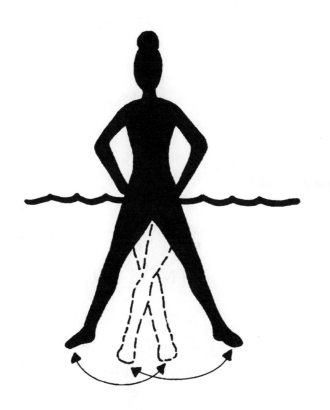

28. LEG SCISSORS:

Jump as you spread your legs apart, jump and cross your legs in the center. Jump and spread your legs apart, jump and cross your legs in the center. Repeat 15 times. (Like "jumping jacks" without the arm movement.)

"They that seldom take pleasure
seldom give pleasure."

Fulke Greville

HEALTH & FITNESS NOTES

29. BIG JUMP:
Gives a gentle cardiovascular workout.
Mobilizes the hip joints.

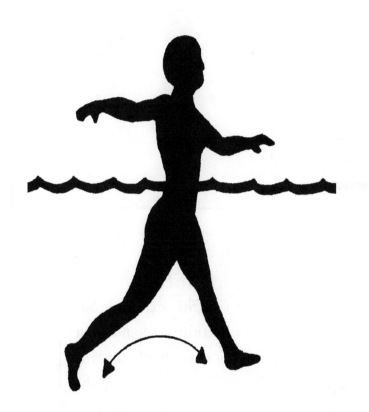

29. BIG JUMP:

Jump stretching Right leg forward and Left leg backward at the same time. Stay in the same spot and jump again, stretch Left leg forward and Right leg backward. Repeat 15 times.

"I pray Thee, O God, that I may
be beautiful within."

Socrates

HEALTH & FITNESS NOTES

30. HIGH KNEES:

Arthritic feet won't like this exercise, but it can be done without landing too hard on the feet. It stretches the lower back, loosens the hip and knee joints. It also works the leg and foot muscles. A nice overall work-out for the lower body.

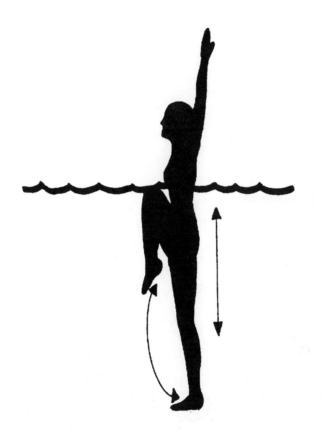

30. HIGH KNEES:

As you jump on your Right foot (flat), bring your Left knee up as high as you can. Jump on your Left foot (flat), bring your Right knee up as high as you can. Repeat 30 times. (Like a majorette marching.)

"*Good books are lengthening and brightening the lives of a multitude of people.*"

Dr. Orison Swett Marden

HEALTH & FITNESS NOTES

31. THE WALK:
Depending on how fast you walk, this can be either a gentle or fairly strenuous cardiovascular workout.

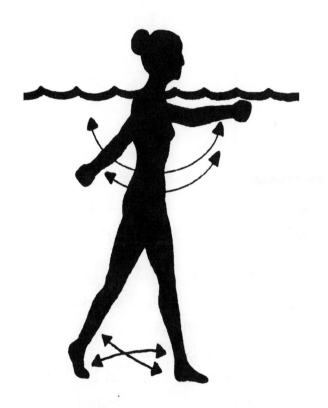

31. THE WALK:

Turn around and walk in a large circle facing the back of the person in front (if you're in a group). As you walk, swing your arms so your Right arm goes forward as your Left leg goes backward; swing your Left arm forward as your Right leg goes backward. Everyone starts with their Right leg. Circle the pool three times to the Right and three times to the Left.

"Love is the poetry of the senses."

Honore de Balzac

HEALTH & FITNESS NOTES

32. HEEL TWIST:
A gentle workout for the lower legs
and ankles.
SIDE NOTE:
Care should be taken so as not to land
hard and strike the heel. It could
fracture or irritate a heel spur.

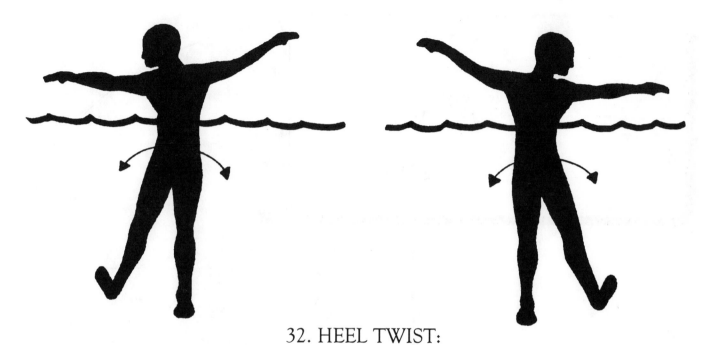

32. HEEL TWIST:

Jump and twist to the Right as you place your Right heel on the bottom of the pool with your toes pointing upward. Jump and twist to the Left as you place your Left heel on the bottom of the pool, with toes pointing up. Pivot to the Right and to the Left. Repeat 30 times. (Like the "Mexican Hat Dance.")

"Excellence is everything.
Because mediocrity is nothing."

James D. Donovan

HEALTH & FITNESS NOTES

33. DOWN SIDES:
Tones the muscles of the sides, reduces
"love handles," and the bulge around
the waist.

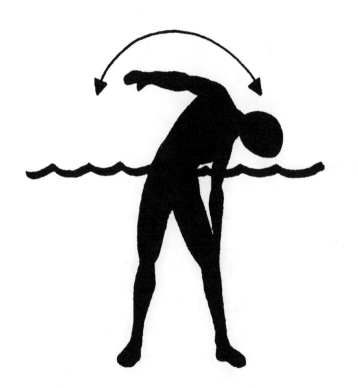

33. DOWN SIDES:

Position your feet shoulder-width apart. With your Right hand, go down the side of your Right leg as far as you can reach, as you bend to the Right. Go down the side of your Left leg with your Left hand as far as you can reach. Alternate Right and Left 30 times.

"*Reading is a pursuit open to everyone, rich and poor alike, and a source of infinite and* unfailing pleasure. "
                                    W.E. Simnett

HEALTH & FITNESS NOTES

34. TOPS OVER:
Tones and shapes the sides and upper, lateral thighs. Trims the waist.

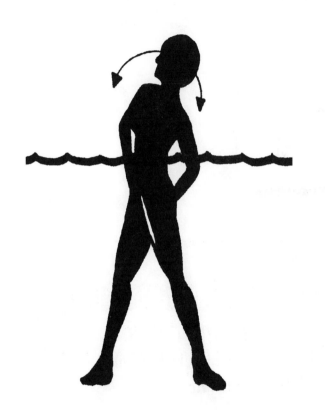

34. TOPS OVER:

With your hands on your hips, bend your shoulders to the Right, bend your shoulders to the Left. Alternate Right and Left. Repeat 30 times. (Keep from hunching and stay tall.)

"*The greatest pleasure I know is
to do a good action by stealth,
and to have it found out by accident.*"

Charles Lamb

HEALTH & FITNESS NOTES

35. HIPS OVER:
This exercise limbers the lower back
and the waist.

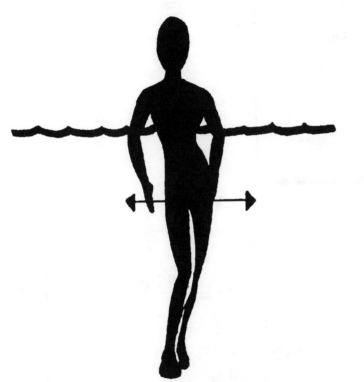

35. HIPS OVER:

Thrust your hips to the Right, push your hips to the Left. Repeat 30 times.

"... the joy of being something and of knowing
that you are advancing is the greatest
of all joys possible to us."

Dr. Judith Powell

HEALTH & FITNESS NOTES

36. BIG HIP CIRCLES:
Mobilizes the lower back muscles
and spine.

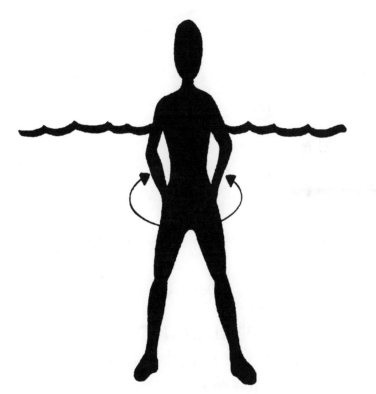

36. BIG HIP CIRCLES:

While standing stationary, roll your hips around in a big circle to the Right 5 times. Roll your hips around in a big circle to the Left 5 times. (Like using a hoola hoop.)

"*When you're good to others,
you are best to yourself.*"

Benjamin Franklin

HEALTH & FITNESS NOTES

37. FIGURE EIGHT:
Mobilizes the lower back muscles
and spine.

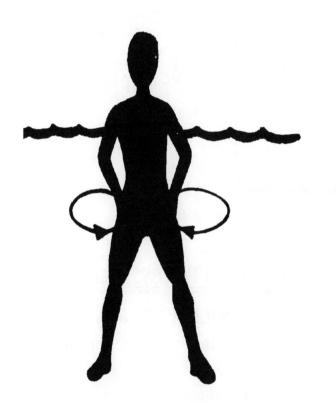

37. FIGURE EIGHT:

Roll your Right hip forward and over to the Right in a semi-circle, roll your Left hip forward to the Left in a semi-circle. You should be making a figure eight. Repeat 30 times. (Like a Hawaiian hoola dance.)

"Let us endeavor to live so that when we come to die even the undertaker will be sorry."

Mark Twain

HEALTH & FITNESS NOTES

38. PULL A STAR:

Tones and stretches muscles of the sides and shoulders. Exercises the shoulder joints.

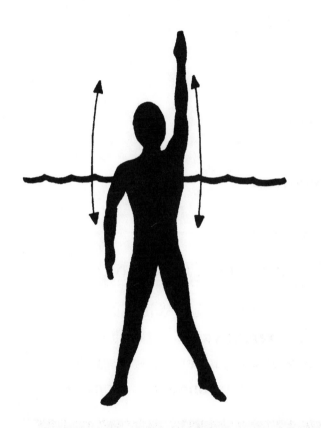

38. PULL A STAR:

Reach way up with your Right arm as if to pull a star down to the water. Do the same with your Left arm. Alternate and repeat 30 times.

"*Great loves should be kept private.*"

Jawaharlal Nehru

HEALTH & FITNESS NOTES

39. STANDING BACK STROKE
This exercise can add flexibility to the upper back and works the muscles of the sides, and upper arms.

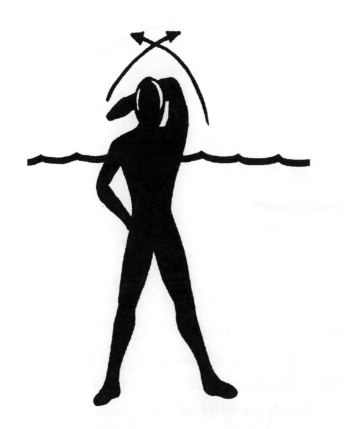

39. STANDING BACK STROKE:

Standing in place, swing your Right arm backward over your head, then swing your Left arm backward over your head. Repeat 30 times.

"A total immersion in life offers the best classroom for learning to love."

Leo Buscaglia

HEALTH & FITNESS NOTES

40. BODY TWIST:

Do this gently. Do not slam from side to side. If done slowly and properly, it will mobilize the lower back.

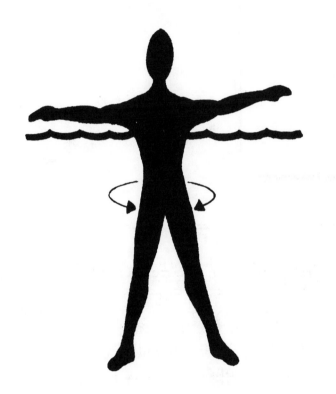

40. BODY TWIST:

Standing with your legs apart, with feet flat, stretch your arms out to the sides just above the water, twist your body to the Right, twist your body to the Left. Repeat 30 times.

"The great use of life is to spend it for something that will out-last it."

William James

HEALTH & FITNESS NOTES

41. KICK OUT SIDEWAYS:
Very good exercise for upper legs and hips.

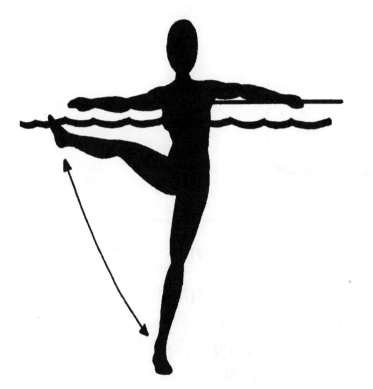

41. KICK OUT SIDEWAYS:

A. Standing in shallow water, hang on to the edge of the pool with your Left hand, kick your Right leg out sideways as high as you can. With a stiff leg, bring your Right leg down to your Left foot. Repeat 10 times.

*"The saying that beauty is but skin deep
is but a skin deep saying."*

John Ruskin

HEALTH & FITNESS NOTES

41. KICK OUT SIDEWAYS:
41B. Strengthens and tones large
muscles of the upper front portion
of the legs.

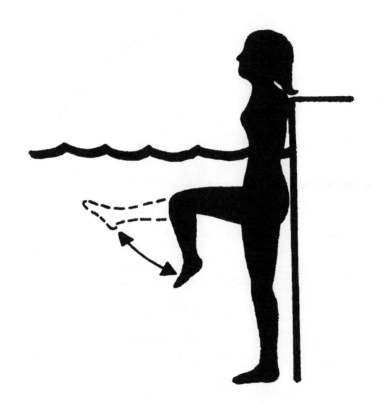

B. While still hanging on the edge of the pool, put your Right knee up facing the center of the pool. Kick your Right leg out from the bent knee position, bring it back, kick out again and bring it back. Repeat 10 times.

"*Charm is a virtue of the heart;
not of the face or figure.*"

John Dryden

HEALTH & FITNESS NOTES

41. KICK OUT SIDEWAYS:
*41C. Strengthens and tones large
muscles of the upper front
portion of the legs.*

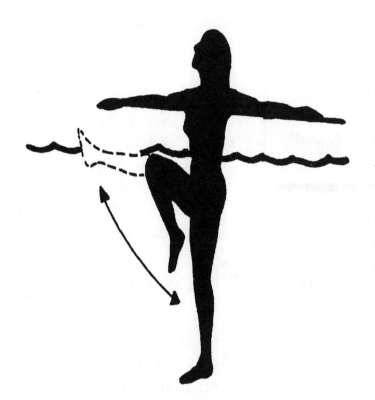

C. Still facing to the Left, kick your Right leg up and out of the water, swing it back down and up in back as far as you can stretch. Repeat 10 times.

❋ Turn around, and do 41A - 41C exercises holding onto the pool this time with your Right hand.

"*Happiness is in the journey,
not in the destination.*"

Dr. Tag Powell

HEALTH & FITNESS NOTES

42. KNEES UP:
Tones and strengthens the upper legs.
It also stretches the lower back.

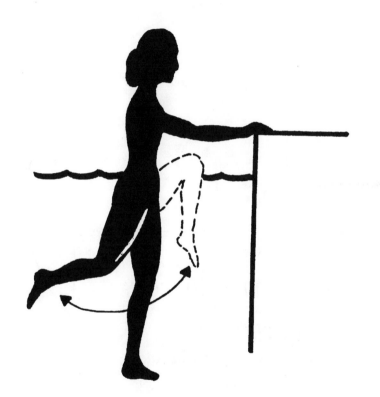

42. KNEES UP:

Facing the wall, hold onto the edge of the pool with both hands, leaving a space between both hands. Bring your Right knee up (toward the surface) and out of the water (as high as you can). Swing it down and swing your leg up in the back, repeat 10 times. Change legs and do the above with your Left knee.

"One should always be peaceful,
even if anger, frustration or heartache
are the ruling emotions of the day."

Alina Nguyen

HEALTH & FITNESS NOTES

43. LEG PUSH:
Exercises the legs and arms.

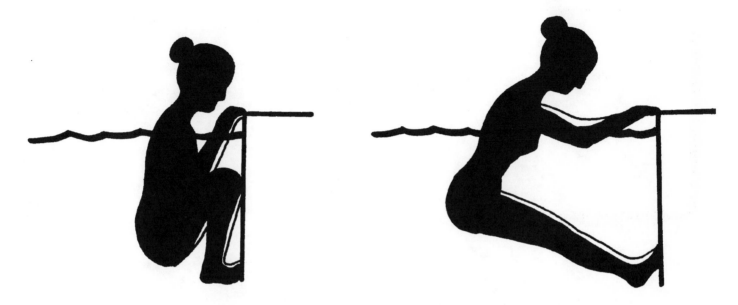

43. LEG PUSH:

Facing the wall of the pool, hang on with both hands. Put both feet on the wall, touch the wall with both knees, push your legs out so both legs are stiff and slightly locked in place. Stay there while you count to 10. Repeat 5 times.

Strengthen and tone with...

DEEP WATER
EXERCISES

"Trust not too much an enchanting face."

Virgil

HEALTH & FITNESS NOTES

1. TWO LEG SWING:
Exercises muscles of the sides and reduces "love handles" on the waist.

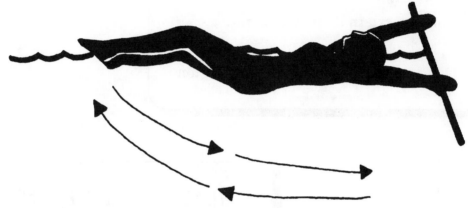

1. TWO LEG SWING:

Hanging onto the edge of the pool, lying on your back near the top of the water, stretch both legs out to the center of the pool. Swing both legs to the Right, touch the Right side of the pool, swing both legs to the Left, touch the Left side of the pool. Repeat 10 times.

"Happiness depends more upon the internal frame of a person's mind, than on the externals in the world."

George Washington

HEALTH & FITNESS NOTES

2. SCISSOR CROSS-OVER:
This exercise tones the front and back of the upper legs and gently strengthens lower abdominal muscles.

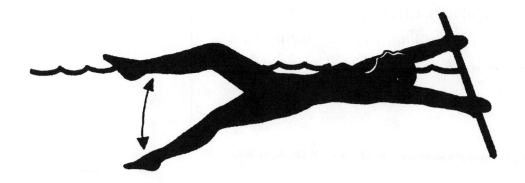

2. SCISSOR CROSS-OVER:

Hanging onto the edge of the pool, lying on your back near the top of the water, stretch both legs out to the center of the pool. Stretch both legs apart as far as you can, bring them back and criss-cross them, swing them apart bring them back and criss-cross them. Repeat 10 times.

"Success is not reached by doing one outstanding thing. Rather, it is the aggregate, the cumulative mass of small tasks and duties done well."

E.R. Brown

HEALTH & FITNESS NOTES

3. FEET UP & DOWN:

Increases mobility of the ankles; stretches calf muscles and muscles of the front lower leg. Pointing the toes up and down as far as possible when doing this exercise also stretches foot muscles for greater flexibility.

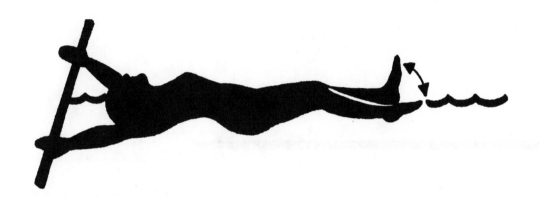

3. FEET UP & DOWN:

Hanging onto the pool, lying on your back with your legs stretched to the center, flip your Right foot up and down from the ankle, flip your Left foot up and down from the ankle, alternating first Right and then Left. Repeat 50 times (each foot).

"*Success is 99% mental attitude.*"

Rousseau

HEALTH & FITNESS NOTES

4. LITTLE CIRCLES:
Adds flexibility to the ankles which decreases the likelihood of muscular sprain or ligament strain.

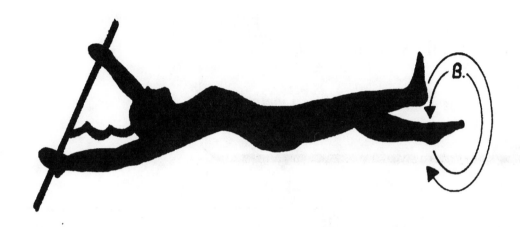

4. LITTLE CIRCLES:

Stay in the same position, lying in the pool on your back, turn both feet inward while making circles 10 times, then make circles turning both feet outward 10 times.

"*We learn only from those we love.*"

Goethe

HEALTH & FITNESS NOTES

5. UP AND OUT:
Tightens lower abdominal (tummy) muscles and flattens the stomach below the belly button. Increases flexibility in the knees and hips. Stretches the lower back.

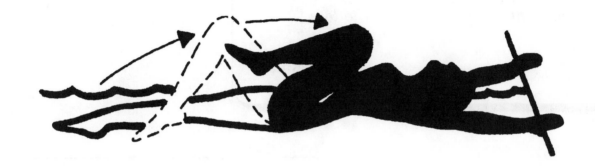

5. UP AND OUT:

Hanging onto the pool on your back near the top of the water, pull both knees up to your chest. Keep your legs together, stretch both legs out to the center, pull them both up to your chest, stretch them out to the center. Repeat 10 times.

125

"When we surrender, we become more loving, and, in the process, we end up showing more of what there is in us to love."

Stela Resnick

HEALTH & FITNESS NOTES

6. TWO LEG CIRCLE SWING:
Gently exercises the abdominal muscles and upper thighs. Mobilizes the lower back, pelvis and knees.

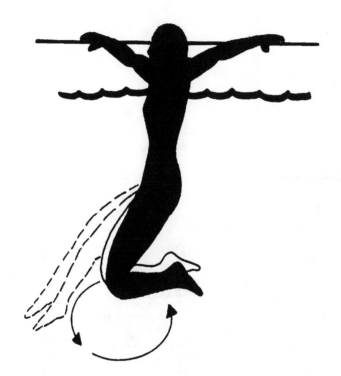

6. TWO LEG CIRCLE SWING:

Hanging vertical, swing both legs around in a circle to your Right. Bend both legs up in back as you go under your derriere, stretch them out as you swing around front, bend them up again as you swing under your derriere. Repeat 5 times, reverse and do 5 more times.

"The word 'impossible' is not in my dictionary."

Napolean Bonaparte

HEALTH & FITNESS NOTES

7. BIG WALK:

Gently stretches and exercises lower back, flattens the stomach and works the front thighs. It will also exercise the hip joints.

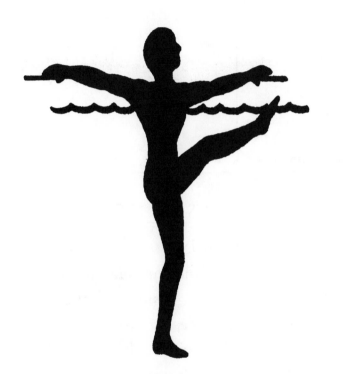

7. BIG WALK:

In a vertical position, hanging onto the side of the pool, do a big walk step. Stretch your Right leg up and out of the water while you stretch your Left leg to the back of the pool, touch your Left heel to the wall, alternating legs as if walking. Repeat 20 times.

"Go to your task with love in your heart, and you will go to it light-hearted and cheerful. Begin; to begin is half the work."

Ausonius

HEALTH & FITNESS NOTES

8. BODY TWIST:

This exercise will thoroughly work out the side muscles and like exercise #1, trims excess fatty tissue in that area.
SIDE NOTE: 50 repeats is excessive, initially. There exists a possibility of overstressing the lower back. It should be slowly worked up to 50 repeats over a period of 1 - 2 weeks.

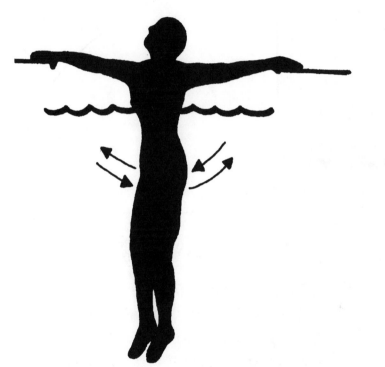

8. BODY TWIST:

Hang onto the pool with arms outstretched. Push away while still hanging on and twist your body to the Right and to the Left. Repeat 50 times.

*"The smiles that inspire the heart
are the kind smiles."*

Samuel Johnson

HEALTH & FITNESS NOTES

9. PENDULUM SWING:
This exercise can add flexibility to the
upper back and works the muscles
of the sides.

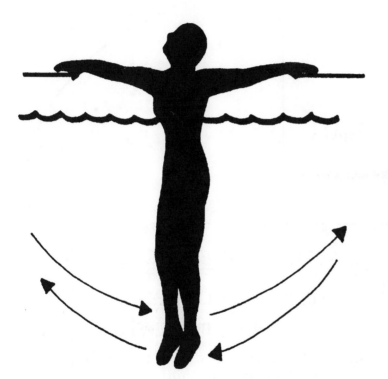

9. PENDULUM SWING:

Hanging onto the pool, with your back against the side, swing your body up to the top of the water on the Left side, swing down toward the bottom of the pool and up to the Right, swing back down and up to the Left side. Repeat 10 times.

*"It is amazing how much both happiness
and efficiency can be increased
by the cultivation of an orderly mind..."*

Aldous Huxley

HEALTH & FITNESS NOTES

10. BOTH LEGS UP:
Great for the abdominal muscles,
stretches the lower back and
exercises the hip joint.

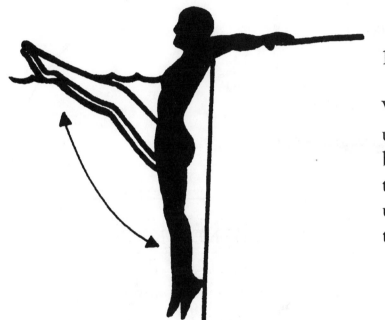

10. BOTH LEGS UP:

With both legs hanging, bring them up together and out of the water. Push both legs down and touch the back of the pool with your heels, bring them up and out of the water, then push them back down. Repeat 10 times.

"... unhappiness is ignorance, and happiness is knowledge."

Paracelsus

HEALTH & FITNESS NOTES

11. FROGGIE:

The froggie is primarily a leg joint exercise, but also tones up the lateral thighs.

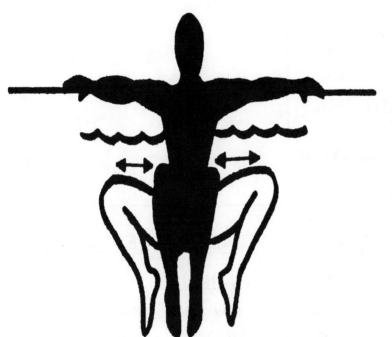

11. FROGGIE:

Put both feet flat on the wall of the pool with knees bent. Bring both knees inward and touch knees together, swing them outward, then bring them inward to touch knees. Repeat 20 times.

"*For, when with beauty we can virtue join,*
We paint the semblance of a form divine."

Matthew Prior

HEALTH & FITNESS NOTES

12. PULL IN BELLY:

A tummy exerciser, and if the derriere
is tightened fully for the full count,
will shape and firm the buns.

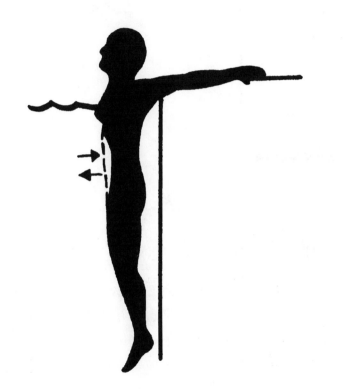

12. PULL IN BELLY:

While hanging vertical in the water, pull your stomach and derriere in tight. Hold to the count of 10, relax. Repeat 10 times.

"Too many waste their energies watching for effects instead of expending these energies upon causes."

Booker T. Washington

HEALTH & FITNESS NOTES

13. CIRCLE ONE LEG:
Emphasizes lower back and hip joint flexibility. Mobilizes the waist.

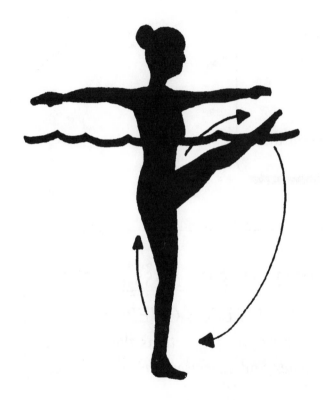

13. CIRCLE ONE LEG:

Make a large circle with your legs, be careful when extending — do it to comfort. Start with your Right leg and go up toward the Right side of the pool. Swing your Right leg out of the water toward the other side of the pool. Bring your Right leg down and across underwater to complete the circle. Repeat 5 times and reverse. Do the same with the Left leg.

"*I believe that we should not forget
how to disagree agreeably
and how to criticize constructively.*"

Margaret Chase Smith

HEALTH & FITNESS NOTES

14. LEGS OVER:
*Firms inner thighs, flattens the stomach,
stretches and exercises the lower back.*

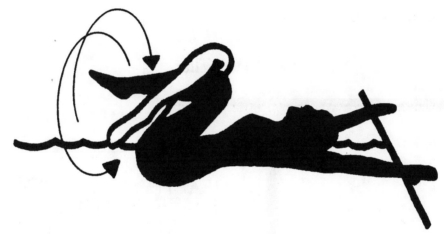

14. LEGS OVER:

Lying on your back with your body slightly in the water, bring your knees up (keep your knees together), swing the Right leg over the Left leg, swing the Left leg over the Right leg. Repeat 30 times.

"True faith is not a fruit of security, it is the ability to blend mortal fragility with the inner strength of the spirit."

Helen Keller

HEALTH & FITNESS NOTES

15. KNEES IN AND OUT:
Tones the lower abdominal region, exercises the hip joints and upper legs, and stretches the lower back.

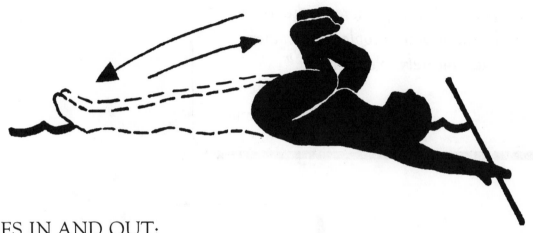

15. KNEES IN AND OUT:

A. Lying near the top of the water, place the soles of your feet flat together. Pull your legs to your chest bending your knees outward, push your legs straight out to the center of the pool keeping your feet together. Repeat 10 times. (Similar to the "froggie," only lying on your back.)

"*The purpose of life is to increase the warm heart. Think of other people. Serve other people sincerely. No cheating.*"

Dalai Lama

HEALTH & FITNESS NOTES

15. KNEES IN AND OUT:
15B. Tones the lower abdominal region, exercises the hip joints, upper legs and stretches the lower back.

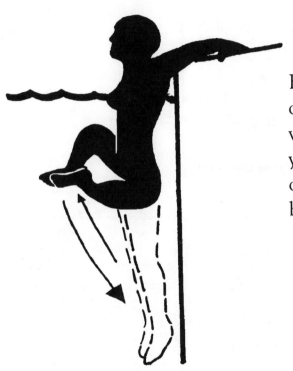

B. Do the same exercise as A., holding onto the pool with your legs hanging vertical, as you pull your legs up bend your knees outward keeping the soles of your feet flat together. Push your legs back down. Repeat 10 times.

"*Kindness costs nothing, we have unlimited storehouses of it.*"

Sir Winston Churchill

HEALTH & FITNESS NOTES

16. HANGING LEGS OVER:
A variation of #14 with the same results.

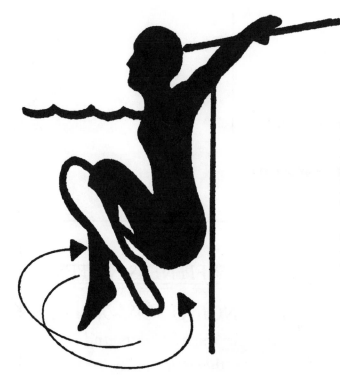

16. HANGING LEGS OVER:

Hanging vertical onto the side of the pool, pull both legs up in a sitting position keeping your knees together. Throw your legs around each other first one leg then the other in a semi-circle. Repeat 50 times.

"Love is liking someone better than you like yourself."

Frank Tyger

HEALTH & FITNESS NOTES

17. HANGING SCISSORS:
Exercises the hip joints and gives them flexibility.

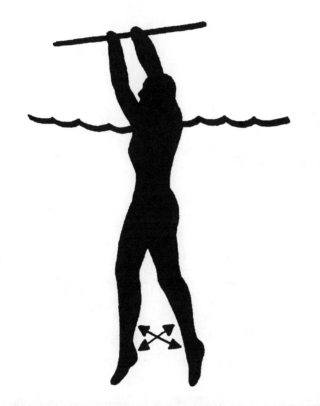

17. HANGING SCISSORS:

Hanging onto the pool in a vertical position, stretch your legs apart. As you bring them together criss-cross them, stretch them apart and criss-cross them again. Repeat 10 times.

"*Whatever you are doing, be happy in it.*"

Samuel Taylor Coleridge

HEALTH & FITNESS NOTES

18. PEDDLE YOUR BIKE:
Stretches lower back, tones the lower
stomach and exercises the hip joints.

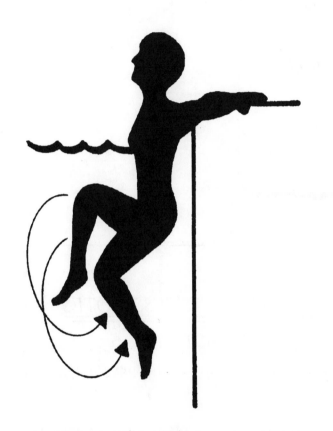

18. PEDDLE YOUR BIKE:

Hang onto the edge of the pool and peddle as if you are peddling your bike. Repeat 50 times.

"*A bright, hopeful, optimistic attitude of mind is essential to your well-being.*"

Robert Green Ingersoll

HEALTH & FITNESS NOTES

19. FAST KICK:
Firms up the fanny and tones the legs.

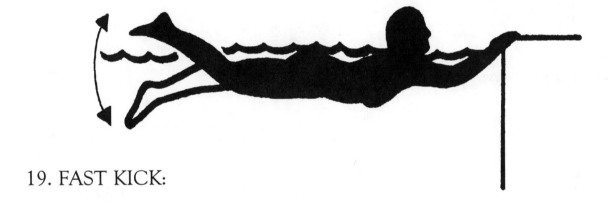

19. FAST KICK:

Lie on your stomach, hang onto the pool and kick 50 times. Turn over on your back and kick 50 more times.

ABOUT THE AUTHOR

Most of Dorothy V. Kelly's life has been spent on or near the water. When the author was three, she learned to swim the "hard" way (and perhaps the only way!). One of her neighbors took Ms. Kelly into deep water to see what she would do if the neighbor were to let go. Of course, her friend remained nearby, but did not actually hold her in the water. The author, on survival instinct, learned to doggie paddle back to shore. Later on, she learned the other strokes by watching swimmers. This experience was Dorothy Kelly's beginning of her love for the water.

Having two daughters in Girl Scouts also helped to further the author's development in water-related activities and led her into water exercising. She became a Scout Leader to spend more time with her children. In this process, Ms. Kelly encouraged them to earn their water safety badges by using the lake which banked their summer cottage. However, obtaining these badges required her children to be taught how to swim by a lifeguard. Finding a person who had the time to accompany them during the summer months became a problem. Therefore, the easiest way was for Dorothy to take the required Junior Life Saving course...her first step towards becoming a trained, certified lifeguard!

Soon-to-follow was the remaining Senior Life Saving course, which Ms. Kelly quickly completed and provided her with an Instructor's Certificate. She used this training to judge her daughters for their water safety badges in swimming, rowing and canoeing. During this time, the author noticed the ease of movement in which water allowed her Girl Scout troop to play and exercise in. The girls had fun, maintained good shapes, and were able to control their activities within a limited area and group.

Along with her Girl Scout leadership, Ms. Kelly also found dancing a lifetime enjoyment. Especially in her younger days, she was part of the Kelly Trio, a dancing vaudeville variety show which she and her brother and sister formed. She later went on to teach dance and put on a great number of shows for schools, P.T.A. clubs and in her retirement park.

After retirement, the author spent her free time in her community's pool. She also tried to maintain an active fitness program, but found that her body had changed with maturity. Therefore, instead of getting out-of-shape, Dorothy gathered a group of friends and adapted her years of experience and training in swimming and dancing to formulate pool exercises.

What the author never realized is that, one day, her easy-to-perform methods would be endorsed by a member of the medical community and published to help ALL senior citizens who want to maintain their physique without actual aerobic exercising!

Ms. Kelly attributes her health and fitness to a lifetime exercise regimen—with safety as priority and fun as the driving force!

VIBRANT HEALTH

The Ultimate Weight, Heart and Health Program
by Clifford T. Stewart, Ph.D. and Lawrence A. Fehr, Ph.D.

Your health is priceless.
What costs are you willing to take?

What does dieting, exercise and proper nutrition mean to you? Starvation? Calorie-counting? Fat in-take levels? Don't be fooled by another gimmick or fad diet. Even exercise is most effective under moderate and safe measures. Your family history and how you think are also part of your level of good or bad health.

Slim down to your perfect fat-to-muscle ratio, and reduce your risk of heart attack, cancer and stress-related diseases. University professors Stewart and Fehr have been advisors on health and nutrition — "telling it like it is" to health professionals and medical doctors for years. Take advantage of their step-by-step guide to healthful living today!

Discover:

* the 8 myths about dieting
* the 10 myths about exercise
* how personality-type and lifestyle affect your health and weight

* the 8 myths about heart disease
* the 12 Stress-Buster techniques
* how to reduce the risks of cancer and heart disease
Includes the "How Long Will You Live?" Test

ISBN 1-56087-015-X, Quality Paperback, 256 pages, includes charts, $12.95 add $3.00 s/h
ISBN 1-56087-071-0, Hardcover with Jacket, includes charts, $21.95 add $3.00 s/h

Write, Phone or FAX For FREE Catalog
Mail to Powell Productions, 11701 S. Belcher Rd., Suite 123, Largo, FL 34643, FAX 813 536-3681 Phone 813 530-0110